C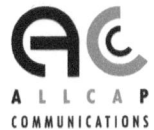VID TALE

A Patient and a Doctor

RABIN CHAKRABORTY

ᴀᴄ
A L L C A P
COMMUNICATIONS

Edited and Designed by Allcap Communications
www.allcap.co.in

Dedicated to

All those who have conquered Covid

&

All those who will bear its scars forever

Contents

Foreword

Covid Tale: A Patient and a Doctor is a remarkable personal narration from a prominent cardiologist; an extraordinary four weeks of his roller-coaster ride in a battle with SARS-CoV-2 (Covid-19). Dr Rabin Chakraborty as a Covid-19 victim shares his feelings with his colleagues and family. He takes us along to share his pain, agony, anxiety and uncertainty.

I can personally identify with his pain and sufferings throughout this story. It brought back the torrent of memories of the weeks I spent with my beloved father during his last days, as he fought with the coronavirus till the very end.

Throughout, Rabin stays true to his two souls, the physician scientist and the brave patient, and he etches both roles with a poet's heart. Accessible to many, this searing personal account helps us to understand and to share the innermost feelings when Covid-19 strikes. It also offers a rare insight into the vulnerability and courage of even an experienced physician when faced with the uncertainty of this uncharted pandemic.

This is a powerful and personal account that engages both the lay person and the physician, offering hope and courage in dealing with this invidious disease.

Suresh Anne
MD FACP FACAAI, FAAAAI
Associate Professor, Division of Allergy and Immunology
Michigan State University
President, Asthma Allergy and Immunology Center
Flint, Michigan USA

Preface

On February 11, 2020, the WHO Director-General, Dr Tedros Adhanom Ghebreyesus, announced that the disease caused by a new coronavirus was "COVID-19", the acronym of "coronavirus disease 2019". Governments around the world desperately tried to control the rampaging virus which brought human life to a near standstill, globally. Eventually this virus spread uninhibitedly like wildfire and on March 11, 2020, WHO declared Covid-19 a pandemic.

The dynamicity and pathophysiology of this virus is mysterious, and its invasion of the human body can be cataclysmic. This upheaval has struck fear in every human soul on this planet. There is colossal uncertainty surrounding Covid-19 with no established treatment or any definite measure to prevent its attack as yet.

I got infected with Covid-19 almost unknowingly, while carrying out my duties as a cardiologist. And it set me on a stormy clinical course, where the outcome hung by a fragile thread. The tumult that this virulent microbe put me through left me shattered and at one point, almost bereft of hope. Yes, even as a medical professional, I did feel helpless and lost at times. But finally, I did emerge from this life-or-death battle, with renewed hope and a deep sense of gratitude.

I strongly felt the need to write down my experience as a Covid-19 victim. My clinical course, the ups and downs of the pathology inside my body, my mental torment, its dynamics are all documented here as a personal diary.

I did feel fear. But fear did not govern me. Amidst fear and apprehension, I remained positive. I kept telling myself that I would win the battle. It is the knowledge, attitude and practice — KAP factor — in any untoward situation that determines the outcome. *Covid Tale: A Patient and a Doctor* is my chronicle as a patient, together with the medical explanation of symptoms and signs of this noxious illness. Some essential facts of Covid-19 have been depicted here.

I am indebted to the Chairman of our hospital, doctors who treated me and specially the critical care team, my consultant pulmonologist, a truly proficient lady, Dr Suresh Anne, immunologist from Michigan, Dr Sanjog Kalra, Covid warrior from Philadelphia, my colleagues of my department, all nurses and technicians, and all category of staff from our hospital and an umpteen number of well-wishers.

Finally, my wife Dr Arundhati Chakraborty, who was also a Covid-19 patient and had a tough time. Despite that, she was always with me through this crisis. My daughter Dr Anindita Chakraborty, a psychiatrist in Michigan, USA, had sleepless nights when both her parents were battling this dreaded disease. She remained stable and constantly rendered her support with positive vibes.

Covid-19 is a disaster. It might have shaken human civilisation of the 21st century to its core, but human society is far too resilient to be beaten by a virus. We will definitely overcome this turmoil and bring our life back to its normal rhythm, to its own melody.

Rabin Chakraborty

Introduction
Kunal Basu

A spectre is haunting our world, the spectre of Covid-19. From expert to lay citizen, it has baffled observers and victims by its rapid spread, giving rise to pervasive panic coupled with sporadic knee-jerk denial. Serving the most severe dose of system shock since the World Wars, it has incapacitated healthcare, national economies and governance in significant parts of the world. It is perhaps fair to say that the impact of Covid-19 has been as cataclysmic if not greater than any other disruption to life in living memory.

Just as medical practitioners have grappled with epidemiology and treatment methods, the virus has spun a web of confusion in the mind of the general public. Conflicting media reports, unverified medical opinion and plain rumour have contributed to at best a partial understanding of the disease, its symptoms and long-term impact on health. It is fair to say that Covid-19 has emerged not simply as a medical but also a sociological phenomenon worthy of investigation.

The challenge, of course, is to examine both the patient's perspective as well as that of the physician in order to arrive at a comprehensive view that reveals as much about the physical experience of the disease as its medical prognosis. It is in this regard that Dr Rabin Chakraborty's book makes a unique and salient contribution.

Expositions on the virus have taken two distinctive

routes thus far: A. Medical reports written by and meant for the consumption of bio-researchers; and B. Journalistic accounts of the terrible sufferings of patients. While both accounts are worthwhile to a spectrum of readers, Dr Chakraborty combines the two through a unique device — report of his own victimhood to the disease and his own assessment of his condition as a physician from the onset of symptoms to their eradication.

Thus, we learn of the circumstances under which he had contracted the virus, how it had manifested its symptoms in him, the critical point at which he chose to be hospitalised (along with his wife) — the full range of bodily sensations described in minute detail. At the same time, his physician's mind kept up an active analysis, monitoring the medical reports, consulting with his attending physicians and, in a sense, charting his own treatment with help from experts.

The effect of this dual view of Covid-19 provides the readers with multiple lenses through which the disease might be examined. It demystifies many commonly held views, corrects misperceptions, but does so with the authenticity of someone who has lived through the experience and borne the brunt of the disease.

Thus, the two voices in the book are both distinct and at the same time blend together to provide a uniform narrative. It is both authentic, and carries the weight of medical expertise. It is a rare example of a physician examining himself and conveying the findings to readers in lucid terms. Once the virus is eliminated and the world comes around to assessing its impact from diverse perspectives, this book will hold its place among the very best in chronicling a most devastating human experience.

Glossary

ARDS	:	Acute respiratory distress syndrome
CCXL, CCL	:	Markers of chemokines (chemicals of inflammation)
CO_2	:	Carbon dioxide
Covid-19	:	Coronavirus of 2019
CRP	:	C-reactive protein (a marker of inflammation)
CT	:	Computerised Tomography
D-dimer	:	A marker of vascular thrombosis
DNA	:	Deoxyribonucleic Acid
ECMO	:	Extracorporeal Membrane Oxygenation
FDA	:	Food and Drug Administration
Ferritin	:	A marker of inflammation
FiO2	:	Pressure of inspired oxygen
HFNO	:	High flow nasal oxygen
ICMR	:	Indian Council of Medical Research
ICU	:	Intensive Care Unit
IL-6, IB, 8, 12	:	Interleukin-6, 1B, 8, 12 (markers of cytokine storm)
LDH	:	Lactate dehydrogenase (a marker of inflammation)
O_2	:	Oxygen
PEEP	:	Positive end-expiratory pressure
PLACID	:	PLAsma Convalescent InDia
PCO2	:	Pressure of carbon dioxide in blood
PO2	:	Pressure of oxygen in blood

RNA   : Ribonucleic Acid
RTPCR   : Reverse transcriptase polymerase chain
             reaction
TrueNAT   : TrueNAT (RNA-dependent RNA polymerase
             gene by microchip) for Covid-19

I

The Beginning

Covid-19, the disease caused by SARS-CoV-2 or the novel coronavirus, is not like the common cold or ordinary flu. This virus is a serious, nasty microbe. It is called corona because of its crown-like appearance. It is a positive single-stranded RNA virus of the COVID family of Corona. It was first identified in December 2019 during the first outbreak in Wuhan, the largest metropolitan city of Hubei province of China.

On February 11, 2020, the WHO Director-General, Dr Tedros Adhanom Ghebreyesus, announced that the disease caused by this new coronavirus was "Covid-19", the acronym of "coronavirus disease 2019". This virus has shaken our planet. Since end-February 2020, this deadly contagion has caused global mayhem and threatened the lives and livelihood of millions.

Right from the medical disaster of the Covid pandemic, to human life, governance, world politics, world economy, working patterns, human attitudes — everything has taken on a new dimension and entered a new paradigm. Deep job losses, prolonged recession and unprecedented debt burdens are creating a political backlash worldwide. More than 75 million people have been affected and close to 1.7 million human lives have been lost by mid-December. That, of course, does not include the death toll from the social tumult the virus has unleashed.

I am a medical practitioner, a cardiologist by profession, taking care of heart patients for 30 years now. I have performed many complex heart procedures not only in India but in several countries all over the world. I have contributed to the advancement in the field of Interventional Cardiology as a doctor, as a postgraduate teacher, as a proctor, as an author of cardiology books, in cardiovascular research, and as international faculty in many cardiovascular meetings. As a cardiologist who cares for the patients' well-being, I used to work relentlessly for at least 12 to 14 hours a day. Even from February till July 2020, my clinical workload did not diminish.

Incubation

On the 30th of July, I was not feeling well. I noticed mild temperature and fatigue, mild aches and a dull pain in my back and my leg muscles, along with a vague unwellness. Enough for that niggle — was I showing early signs of the noxious corona bug?

With defiance as my default setting, I took some paracetamol. The fever went down in 30 minutes. I felt a lot better and forgot about it. The next day I was fine and I went to the hospital. I had been seeing patients taking all standard precautions like using a sanitiser, wearing the N-95 mask, and gloves. Social distancing, however, was not possible in real terms as being a doctor I have to examine patients properly. Three patients I saw were Covid-19 positive, which I came to know later.

After two days, I again had mild fever, a general feeling of malaise, occasional dry cough, but no shortness of breath. I continued to remain in denial mode, as if the virus might affect others but not me. Nevertheless, a nagging suspicion nudged me towards a Covid-19 test, an RTPCR (rapid test for polymerase chain reaction), after two days — the Monday after the weekend. On Tuesday morning around 5am, I suddenly noticed that my wife, Arundhati, had high-grade fever with severe chill and rigor.

That was a true wake-up call for me. I was convinced that the deadly virus had invaded us, stealthily.

Day 1

It was time to act. We reached the tertiary care hospital in Kolkata, to which I am attached as the Senior Vice Chairman and Head of Cardiology Services, around 10.30am. I requested for the nasal and throat swabs for RTPCR and TrueNAT (RNA-dependent RNA polymerase gene by microchip) for Covid-19, virus and blood tests.

We were isolated in a twin-sharing room. Swabs were taken from the back of oral and nasal cavities. Blood tests were done. Arundhati and I were anxiously waiting for the reports, which came after around eight hours. We were both Covid-19 positive, confirmed by both TrueNAT and RTPCR methods.

Clearly, I was not invincible.

My white cell count was high, lymphocytes were low.

My C-reactive protein (CRP) was high and liver functions were deranged. Lactate dehydrogenase (LDH) and serum ferritin were mildly raised and D-dimer, Interleukin-6 (IL-6) were also elevated indicating that it was more than just being Covid-positive. There was a virus load within me and Arundhati, called viraemia. Our body system had been attacked by the Covid-19 virus and the body had initiated reactions to this invasion. This demanded hospital admission.

I requested the hospital that I be excused for a night so that I could go back home, with the promise that the following morning both of us would come in for admission. The hospital authority, reluctantly, agreed to let us go for the night.

We came home. My 87-year-old mother was there. We made arrangements for her care with the domestic help along with her food, medicines, financial support, etc. My mother was doing well; all precautions were being taken for the last four months. I explained our medical condition to her and that both Arundhati and I needed to be hospitalised from the next morning for at least two to three weeks. I did not sleep well that night.

Day 2

The next morning, Arundhati and I went to the hospital and got admitted. We were straightway taken to the radiology department for a CT scan of the chest. The consultant in charge and the Chairman of the hospital were there in the

CT suite. They were very supportive. My CT chest revealed Covid-19 patches on both sides of lung bases and at the back extending up to mid chest. The left side had more involvement than the right. I was not too breathless at that time. Arundhati's CT chest result was better; she had rather mild Covid pneumonia. Within 15 minutes, we were in private rooms on the sixth floor of the hospital. The Covid-19 virus might have entered through our nose or mouth. It was inside us and growing slowly, causing fever and flu-like symptoms. As a further consequence, there was lung involvement.

II

Viraemia

Corona viruses are a large family of viruses which may cause illness in animals or humans. In humans, several corona viruses are known to cause respiratory infections ranging from the common cold to more severe diseases such as Middle East Respiratory Syndrome (MERS) and Severe Acute Respiratory Syndrome (SARS). This new virus, SARS-CoV-2, and disease, Covid-19, were unknown before the outbreak began in Wuhan, China, in December 2019. Covid-19 is now a pandemic affecting almost all countries in the world.

Viruses are infectious agents of small size and simple composition that can multiply only in living cells. All viruses contain a nucleic acid, either DNA (deoxyribonucleic acid) or RNA (ribonucleic acid), and several RNA viruses should not even be considered organisms since they are not free-living. They require a host cell, and thus these viruses need to elude the host immune defence system to infect its cells in order to reproduce, replicate and survive.

People can catch Covid-19 from others who have the virus. The disease spreads primarily from person to person through small droplets from the nose or mouth, which are expelled when a person with Covid-19 coughs, sneezes, or speaks. These droplets are relatively heavy, do not travel far and quickly sink to the ground. People can catch Covid-19 if they breathe in these droplets from a person infected with the virus. It is, therefore, important to stay at least 2 metres away from others because the mechanism of transmission of this novel coronavirus involves air droplets emanating from a patient.

These droplets can land on objects and surfaces around the infected person such as tables, doorknobs and handrails where they stay for at least four hours. People can become infected by touching these objects or surfaces and then touching their eyes, nose or mouth.

The virus mainly harbours in the rear side of the oral and nasal cavities, oropharynx and nasopharynx respectively. There, it replicates and grows. During this stage of virus replication there may be no symptoms or mild flu-like symptoms, fever, dry cough, muscle pain, and a general feeling of being unwell. Most common symptoms of Covid-19 are fever, dry cough, and tiredness. Other symptoms that are less common and may affect some patients include headache, body ache, nasal congestion, conjunctivitis, sore throat, diarrhoea, loss of taste or smell, rash on skin or discoloration of fingers or toes. These symptoms are usually mild and begin gradually. Some people become infected but do not display symptoms. They are often super-spreaders.

Most people (around 80 per cent) recover from the disease without requiring hospital treatment. Around one out of every five patients with Covid-19 becomes seriously ill and develops difficulty in breathing, incessant cough, severe hypoxaemia. Older people and those with coexisting medical problems such as high blood pressure, heart and lung diseases, diabetes, or cancer are at higher risk (as high as 20%) of developing serious infirmity secondary to Covid-19.

During the early infection phase or Phase 1), the virus multiplies inside the body and is likely to cause mild symptoms not dissimilar to those of the common cold. Many a time it may remain unnoticed or be mistaken for a simple flu. Covid-19 can not only cause prolonged episodes of cough, cold, high fever and breathing difficulties that do not subside with conventional medication, it is also a highly infectious disease. It can spread from a sick person or from an asymptomatic carrier to a healthy individual through mere close contact.

This is the time when most people do not realise that it could be Covid-19 viraemia. With a delay in diagnosis and treatment, the virus continues to grow and multiply inside the body up to 10 days, then subsides. And in one out of five patients, the more serious Phase 2 of the disease, the cytokine storm, sets in and complications begin.

This virus, unlike many other respiratory viruses, seldom causes severe pneumonia or primary infection of the lung. The Covid-19 story is somewhat different. The viral load can be ascertained from the throat and nasal swabs and probably from chest CT pictures. Viral load or the degree of viraemia may or may not have a direct correlation with the clinical course and complications of this disease. But it is not easy to ascertain the virus load clinically and its assessment even by nasal or oral swab has fallacies. Furthermore, the clinical course of Covid-19 infection is quite unpredictable — especially when patients seek medical attention late. Therefore, anyone can catch Covid-19 and become seriously ill without much warning signs.

People of all ages who experience fever and/or cough associated with difficulty in breathing or shortness of breath, chest pain/pressure should seek medical attention immediately. Even at the early stage when there is fever, flu-like symptoms along with loss of taste or smell, it is advisable to alert a healthcare provider or go to a medical facility at the earliest. The person can then be tested and undergo thorough investigations, and be directed to a Covid hospital.

In these precarious times of the sweeping spread of this lethal disease, the best way to remain protected and disease-free is prevention. In case there are early symptoms, immediate check-up, testing for Covid-19, other blood tests and commencement of medication at the stage of viraemia are of paramount importance.

III

Days 2, 3, 4 and 5

After the CT chest, we were taken to the sixth floor and lodged in private rooms — two adjacent ones with a glass door in between. Nurses in PPE (personal protection equipment) checked our vitals. Doctors, nurses, technical staff, housekeeping, everyone looked the same. Everyone was in PPE. Their faces and eyes could not be seen clearly. No human touch was felt as they handled us with gloves. Nevertheless, all of them were very courteous and caring.

Being a doctor, I know how tough it is to remain inside the PPE for more than eight hours at a stretch. You feel awfully hot and suffocated. You can't eat or drink properly or even go to the washroom. But you must be available when any patient asks for you. You need to remember everything of every patient — from vital parameters to the timings of medicines. There were 11 patients in the Covid ward on the sixth floor. My thoughts turned to how these healthcare workers were serving them round the clock during this time of crisis.

Has anyone, including the patients that they care for, ever considered what it is like to be a healthcare worker in the time of a pandemic? Many of them are working far away from their homes. Has anyone really tried to understand their mental state? Their sincerity towards their duty, however, is unflinching and extraordinary. A silent feeling of gratitude swept through me. Outside, a gentle drizzle made the weather nice and comfortable.

Nurses started recording temperature, blood pressure, and oxygen saturation. A few more blood tests — complete blood count, inflammatory markers like CRP, ferritin, kidney and liver function tests, coagulation parameters, D-dimer, and IL-6 — were done instantaneously. These were markers of cell destruction of vital organs and possible predictors of clinical outcome. We were prescribed some medicines, which would probably be dispensed after lunch.

My viral load was heavy as per the RTPCR test and also from the CT chest findings. The virus might have entered around a fortnight ago and the viraemia had probably progressed silently inside my body over a period of six to seven days — the time when I was in denial. I did have some comorbid issues like mild hypertension, mild asthma, and I was 64 years old. I did not have diabetes, heart disease, or any other chronic illness

In the hospital, on Days 2 and 3, I felt no real distress. I walked around the corridor of the ward four to five times every day, for 10 to 15 minutes each time. There was no fever, no breathing discomfort, the oxygen saturation was more than 97 per cent in room air. On Day 3, my consultant was very happy to see me comfortable. He assured me that I might be able to go home in the next two days if everything continued to remain stable.

However, my blood reports showed no improvement in CRP, IL-6. Same with the D-dimer. Deep inside,

I was perturbed.

Day 4 was also rather uneventful. During the daytime I had a mild temperature of 99.5°F. I was on an antibiotic. There was an occasional mild dry cough but no breathlessness. My investigational reports, however, were pointing towards a clinical condition that might compel me to stay longer in the hospital. Another set of blood tests was done. Psychologically I was disturbed, although I did not articulate that.

As night approached, I had a premonition that the ride ahead might not be as smooth as it had been so far; I might develop complications and might even be very close to fatality. But, after fighting hard, I would possibly come out of a very critical condition. Around 2am, I wrote a poem about myself and mentioned that even if I had to leave this planet, it won't be this time. I would survive this and was sure to continue to live in this beautiful world. The omen won't take me away, I penned down defiantly.

Next day, Day 5, my condition was stable. I went to the washroom. My vitals were stable. Oxygen saturation was around 95-96 per cent. I had a good appetite; I was walking in the corridor for at least 10 to 15 minutes two to three times with not much discomfort. The blood test results of Day 4 came in. There was a drop of lymphocytes, liver enzymes remained high, CRP, D-dimer, IL-6 were going up. Clearly, something was not right.

From the evening, I noticed that my oxygen saturation was not going above 92-93 per cent even at rest. More so when I was returning from the washroom. Oxygen saturation in the pulse oximeter was at times less than 90 per cent. I was, however, not feeling much distress; I was rather comfortable.

This is classical "happy hypoxia" or more accurately hypoxaemia, which means significant drop of oxygen in the blood. It is a characteristic of the coronavirus infection that oxygen saturation may drop but the patient may not feel much distress initially. In an otherwise normal person once the saturation goes below 94 per cent, then clearly the oxygen utilisation of organs such as lungs, brain, heart, kidney, liver is dropping and that may even be the beginning of organ failure. In any other medical illness, patients get symptoms such as breathlessness, weakness, fatigue and there is a progressive slide downhill as the oxygen saturation drops below 90 per cent.

However, in Covid-19 infection, there is a paradox. Oxygen saturation may even drop below 90, to life-threatening levels, but the patient remains steady.

Being a doctor, I was familiar with "happy hypoxia", although I was experiencing it for the first time. I requested the nursing in-charge and started taking oxygen by nasal cannula, 4 litre/minute. The oxygen saturation went up to 96-97 per cent. I felt a lot better. The night passed without any trouble. Was I turning a corner? Well, read on....

IV

Happy Hypoxia

Sometimes patients with hypoxia don't experience shortness of breath even though their oxygen levels have dropped to a dangerous point. This phenomenon is referred to as "silent" or "happy" hypoxia, where the body has oxygen saturation below 90 per cent but the person can still breathe normally and does not have any symptoms. Happy hypoxia occurs in coronavirus patients when there are areas of the lung where ventilation is quite normal but there may be enough disease in other areas — like base and back of lungs — with lower oxygen levels. These patients will still have good enough lung function in terms of how the lungs move — they're able to adequately blow off (expiration) their carbon dioxide (CO_2), so they don't develop shortness of breath.

This "happy hypoxia" condition could be due to the brain's insensitivity towards low oxygen content of the blood. Pulmonologists from Loyola University of Chicago, USA, theorised this. The respiratory centre of the brain fails to send signals to the cerebral cortex that with the fall of oxygen content in the blood the body needs to have more ventilation and thus the breathing rate should go up. From the outside, the patient looks comfortable but actually is sinking fast. In addition, there is fluid accumulation inside the lung's micro air spaces, alveoli, leading to micro collapse of the lung. Cells of lung blood vessels are also damaged, leading to micro-thrombosis.

Low oxygen in the blood, hypoxaemia, with relatively low level of blood CO_2 and much more complex mechanisms preclude the manifestations of symptoms of hypoxaemia. A state of "happy hypoxia" sets in, which out of the blue may become an ominous sign of criticality.

Cytokine Storm/Chemokine Storm

The term "cytokine storm" has become increasingly used when we talk about the Covid-19 infection. It is likely that the widespread use of this term is related with its rather immediate meaning, which actually recalls the role of the immune system in producing an uncontrolled and generalised inflammatory response. Unlike many viral pneumonias, the Covid-19 virus does not cause direct pneumonia by directly infecting the lung parenchyma tissue. It initiates violent immune reactions in the host that release chemicals and stimulate the cellular adhesions. The inner cells of blood vessels lose integrity, leading to micro-thrombosis. There is inflammation and fluid collection inside lung tissue. All these cause a picture like pneumonia, damage of lung blood vessels. Lungs then collapse, as if killed by the microbe.

In simpler terms, severe Covid pneumonia does not mean that a huge load of virus has invaded the lung and caused direct inflammation. It means some patients infected with the Covid-19 virus develop an overreaction of the immune system, which triggers a syndrome called cytokine storm.

This storm has a direct correlation with complications like complex chest pathology, severe hypoxaemia, fast heart rate, low blood pressure, cardiac arrhythmias, myocarditis, kidney injury, liver damage, even brain stroke or acute neuropsychiatry feature. Complications may lead to fatality.

Not the virus itself, but the body's own immune cells and the body's own chemicals are killing its own organs. The duration of such a storm is unpredictable, unknown, intriguing and mysterious.

Since the first reports on Covid-19, it seemed clear that severe lung damage leading to very low level of oxygen, known as acute respiratory distress syndrome (ARDS), accounts for a significant number of deaths among infected patients and that ARDS should be regarded as the hallmark of complex immune-mediated clinical consequence in Covid-19 infection.

ARDS is a devastating condition, with an estimated mortality of nearly 40 per cent. There is presence of infiltrates in both lungs and severe hypoxemia. The inflammatory injury to the lung alveoli-capillary membrane results in increased lung permeability. Protein-rich inflammatory fluids accumulate inside lung micro air spaces, make the lung stiff and white, leading to severe respiratory failure.

The materials called surfactants that keep the micro lung spaces known as pulmonary alveoli open, tend to dry up, as a result of which surface tension is lost leading to the collapse of alveoli. Therefore, the available lung area for exchange of oxygen and carbon dioxide from air gets significantly diminished. In Covid-19, such a thing begins mostly at the lower part and back of the lungs. Along with these, there is lung blood vessel damage, known as vasculopathy, causing small vessel thrombosis and leading to complex lung thrombosis. Such coagulation defects and blood vessel thrombosis are unique to the Covid-19 infection. The cells lining the blood vessels of the human body are affected. In lungs, such inflammation of blood vessels results in thrombosis. However, worldwide, medical specialists took at least three to four months to recognise this.

The entire pathological process of the Covid-19 infection is really complex and many physicians did not comprehend all this in the early stages of the pandemic. That might explain why there was higher mortality in the initial months in Italy, Spain, the UK, and the USA. Behaviour of the Covid-19 infection and its trajectory were quite inexplicable then, and to some extent even now.

Increased circulating levels of pro-inflammatory cytokines, like Interferon γ, interleukin (IL, 1B, IL-6, IL-12) and chemokines (CXCL10, and CCL2) are associated with pulmonary inflammation and extensive lung involvement. More importantly, the so-called "cytokine storm" has emerged as the critical factor driving a more severe clinical course. All these cytokines in turn attract and release chemokines. These are the main culprits in the Covid-19 infection and its complications. There is a defect in oxygen utilisation and metabolism of all vital organs. Oxygen-carrying capacity of haemoglobin gets significantly compromised and all essential organs such as lung, heart, liver, kidney, gut and brain suffer severe oxygen deficiency, which may eventually lead to multi-organ failure.

This concept originated from the observation that Covid-19 patients requiring ICU admission displayed higher concentrations of cytokines and chemokines such as CXCL10, CCL2 and TNF-α as compared to those in whom the infection was less severe and who did not require ICU admission. In fact, before this Phase 2, the virus load starts diminishing. More than the virus itself it is the cytokine storm, a reaction of the body's own immune system "attacking" the body, which may prove lethal.

Chemokine storm is the after-effect of a cytokine storm. As the body reacts against the Covid-19 virus, cytokines are released in abundance by the immune system. This in turn triggers the chemical or chemokines to be released. Consequently, a lot of cellular elements such as leukocytes and thrombocytes become very adhesive, get clumped and cause microvascular thrombosis, cellular inflammation of the organs such as lungs, causing pneumonitis, in heart muscles causing myocarditis, vasculitis in the brain, gastrointestinal tract, etc. There could be kidney involvement and nerve involvement. Acute lung failure, acute heart rhythm disorders, heart failure, brain stroke, acute psychiatry features may get manifested. Multiple organs are affected progressively and unpredictably. Gradually, the patient starts sinking.

[v]

Day 6

In the morning I felt a little better. There was no fever. I had a mild cough but breathing was effortless, blood pressure was 134/78 mmHg, oxygen saturation was 96 per cent. Blood samples were drawn in the morning. Blood reports came by 11am and showed rising levels of C-reactive protein, LDH, ferritin, D-dimer, even elevated IL-6. All these markers had been showing a progressive rise since admission, indicating that my body's immune system had started reacting violently against the Covid-19 virus, releasing toxic chemicals. Although, subjectively, I was not feeling too bad. What a paradox!

Clearly, I was now in Phase 2 of the Covid-19 infection — that is, the cytokine/chemokine storm. I knew this phase was uncharted territory shrouded in mystery, and often treacherous. I volunteered to remain on at least 4 litre/minute of oxygen for the entire day. Even then, while walking out of the washroom or even after lunch or dinner, I was feeling breathless. My breathing rate was 28-30/minute, pulse rate was 96/min.

That happy hypoxia was probably weakening. I started showing clear symptoms. Oxygen deficiency in my body was setting in. Blood haemoglobin was not carrying adequate oxygen to my vital organs. Intravenous Remdesivir was started, hoping to spark some improvement. The nagging doubt I had was, if I was in Phase 2, when the viraemia might be passing off, how would Remdesivir, an antiviral drug, help at this stage?

By night, I could feel that I was no longer in the same condition as the previous night. Saturation was dropping to 90 to 92 per cent despite being on oxygen. Some doctors came from critical care around midnight. They changed the cannula to an oxygen mask with a flow rate of 6-8 litre/hour. A bedside monitor was fixed with continuous monitoring of pulse, oxygen saturation, respiration rate and blood pressure. A senior nurse was stationed near my bed and she was ever vigilant about my condition.

The nurses in the ward were excellent. All of them were in PPE, taking very special care of me — at the risk of getting infected. Were they not thinking of their families and themselves? Their commitment to service was amazing. I bowed my head and saluted them silently. The whole night I had some breathlessness even on oxygen and did not sleep well. The nurse next to me was very supportive. Perhaps her main concern was that should my condition deteriorate I might need to be transferred to the critical care unit during the night.

[VI]

Hypoxia and Hypoxaemia

The virus that causes Covid-19 is new to humans and as a result its virulence and disease trajectory are unclear. Treatment has developed along the way as the pandemic has progressed. In all countries, since the disease was first identified, it has been accepted that a high number of patients with severe Covid-19 disease develop acute respiratory distress syndrome (ARDS) and require respiratory support. There may be low oxygen in the blood, hypoxaemia, low oxygen in arterial blood, as seen in the blood gas reports (PaO2 < 60 mmHg), without increase in carbon dioxide hypocapnia PCO2 < 35mm Hg (hypercapnia or carbon dioxide retention inside the body). This is defined as Type 1 respiratory failure. In Covid-19, often there is hypoxaemia together with hypocapnia (arterial PCO2 < 35 mmHg).

Hypoxia is low oxygen in the body tissue at cellular level. Hypoxia is a clinical situation when oxygen saturation is less than 93 per cent by oximeter. It is hypoxaemia, arterial blood oxygen less than 60 mmHg, that is more important. These patients commonly have fast breathing known as tachypnoea, increased use of accessory muscles, fast heart rate (tachycardia), pale and cold limbs, sweating, confusion, agitation or reduced level of consciousness, and blue skin, called cyanosis. When the oxygen content in the blood is low, organs suffer critical oxygen shortage. Vital organs such as heart, lungs, brain, liver, kidneys start failing.

VII

Day 7

In the morning the discomfort was less; I was still on 6 litre/minute of oxygen. I managed to go to the washroom but suffered breathing difficulty. I had my breakfast. By 10am I was experiencing increased breathing difficulty along with cough and chest spasm. Oxygen flow was increased to 8 litre/minute and that brought some respite. But I could feel my general sense of awareness going down. I was feeling dull and apathetic, losing strength, feeling as if I would collapse any moment. Intravenous saline was started. By 1pm, I was breathing fast with palpitation and my mental condition was cloudy. Oxygen saturation was 82 per cent and blood pressure was 94/60 mmHg with pulse rate of 130/minute.

Clearly, I was sinking.

My consultant rushed into the room and immediately decided to transfer me to the ICU. A big oxygen cylinder was brought in. It was turned on at a very high flow. The saturation went up to 96 per cent. I could see Arundhati looking completely helpless, anxiety writ large, as I was being wheeled out of the ward on a trolley towards intensive care.

I was equally unsure about my fate at that time. However, I was committed to complying with my consultant's decision. Everything was being done with the best intention. The attending nurse was very supportive, and her words sounded encouraging to me. She accompanied me till the ICU.

Transfer to Intensive Care Unit

I was taken to the ICU. I was developing acute respiratory distress syndrome and would require respiratory support. Blood gas analysis showed definite Type 1 respiratory failure with low oxygen content in blood (less than 55 mmHg) and low carbon dioxide (less than 30 mmHg). A portable chest X ray was brought in. It was bad. The left lung had become almost white with partial white shadows of the right lung up to mid chest. There was a discussion about early intubation. Invasive mechanical ventilation was being considered. However, the pulmonologists and the critical care team decided to initiate some kind of non-invasive ventilation with high flow nasal oxygen (HFNO).

This is a device which runs on a motor propeller and delivers high oxygen flow — 15 to 20 litre/min of 60-70 per cent, guided by sterile saline flow. It tries to open up lung alveoli (micro spaces) and prevents lung collapse by opening up the trapped or micro collapsed lung alveoli. As there is a collection of inflammatory materials inside the lung tissue, such rapid clearance by HFNO will keep the lung tissue functioning and thus oxygenation for lung ventilation will continue.

My critical care consultant explained how the advantage of using HFNO was humidification of oxygen to prevent dehydration of the airway passages. The high flow rates can be used to provide carbon dioxide "washout". This would stop accumulation of carbon dioxide inside the body, which might cause respiratory depression.

My consultant pulmonologist was a very competent lady doctor with accomplished skill and wisdom. She insisted that by all means I must remain on HFNO and must lie down on my chest, popularly known as the prone position. But it is not easy to tolerate such high flow through wide-bore nasal cannula. The tubes of this device are wide bore and sit very tight on the nostrils. It was uncomfortable and cumbersome but at that stage it would function as my lifeline.

I was getting HFNO at 10 litre/minute of 60 per cent oxygen initially. Arterial blood gas was done two to three times daily to monitor the oxygen and carbon dioxide content in the blood. My pulmonologist very clearly explained to me the importance of HFNO and reassured me that I might not require invasive ventilation, if I strictly adhered to HFNO-guided oxygen support and maintained at least 12-14 hours of prone position.

She also explained to me that in prone position, the lungs at the back and the lower parts would expand more, which meant more ventilation. In Covid-19 infection there is severe hypoxaemia, which means oxygen-carrying capacity of haemoglobin goes down significantly. In addition, there was inflammation of lung tissue, increased inflammation of lung vasculature and the tissue at the interface between blood vessels and lung tissue were also affected. There was ARDS. In such cases, functional lung volume significantly diminishes, progressively. But in Covid-19 infection, the lung might not shrink significantly. In a majority of Covid-19 patients, there could be many white shadows or patches in the lungs, more so on the back and lower side and mid chest region causing respiratory distress, incessant hacking cough, bronchospasm and drop of oxygen saturation.

Despite ARDS, the majority of Covid-19 lungs are not small and stiff ("baby lung") but have near-normal compliance and are therefore unlikely to benefit from high positive end-expiratory pressure (PEEP) at the initial stage.

My critical care consultant and pulmonologist explained that they preferred not to go for mechanical ventilation at this stage. After HFNO, I became much more alert and could comprehend what they were saying. Early introduction of mechanical ventilation was not going to be helpful. Lung volume might continue to hold for some time and that was the reason why HFNO and prone position were mandatory rather than straightway subjecting me to mechanical ventilation. In 80% patients on ventilator, it is tough to bring them off the ventilator and often prognosis remains guarded.

What happens with Covid-19 is that ventilation in the lung and blood flow in the lung are significantly mismatched in a cytokine storm. The infection affects the lungs badly, mostly the base and back — as in my case. The prone position improves the blood circulation and ventilation or oxygenation of blood and it also prevents micro collapse of the functioning lung tissue. Chances of collapse may be minimised and HFNO would try to keep the micro lung tissue opened up and thus prevent collapse of the lung.

My pulmonologist clearly explained to me that ventilation in my case would be challenging as there were multiple pathologies like lung inflammation, vascular damage, even some fluid collection. I must have a good trial of HFNO and at least 14-18 hours of prone position along with medication. She was very clear in her plan of treatment. I was convinced and I promised to myself that whatever might be the outcome I must comply with her advice hundred per cent.

HFNO was going at a very high rate and I was flat on the bed on my chest. By this time drugs like Remdesivir, some antibiotics, and saline were going through my veins. Arterial blood gas analysis every eight hours, blood biochemistry twice and continuous monitoring of all vital parameters were on. Blood reports were strongly suggestive of rising cytokines such as IL-6 and other parameters were also progressively rising. My pulmonologist advised plasma therapy. In her experience, many Covid-19 patients improved with plasma transfusion.

The World Health Organization (WHO) has supported the use of HFNO in Covid-19 patients with ARDS. But it has recommended close monitoring for clinical deterioration, rising breathing rate, increased breathlessness and progressive drop of oxygen. These indicate no improvement with HFNO, which could require emergency intubation. Mechanical ventilation, in turn, increases the risk of complex infections and other complications of invasive ventilation.

While HFNO was on, one unit of plasma A-positive was commenced hoping that my condition would improve. By then, I had no clue. I was mentally in too cloudy a state to comprehend these details. I tolerated the plasma transfusion well; there was no adverse reaction. I felt less breathless and the exhaustion seemed reduced to some extent. It was, of course, too early to expect any clinical improvement within a few hours of plasma therapy.

Day 8

With HFNO and prone position there was some improvement clinically, but the blood gas reports were not good, the oxygen content was low. I was breathless. Respiratory rate was 30/minute, a hacking cough continued with spasm in the chest. Remdesivir and convalescent plasma therapy did not help me much. I was taken for another CT chest. It showed that lung damage had increased significantly, especially in the left lung. Intravenous Remdesivir, anticoagulants like Enoxaparin and Apixaban were being continued. Liver enzymes were elevated. An opinion came in about intravenous Tocilizumab therapy at this point. But looking at the rising liver enzymes and doubtful benefits as per medical literature at that stage, it was not commenced.

Being a doctor, I realised that I was steadily sliding downhill. More so after knowing that my lungs were worse on the last CT scan and the blood gas was showing worsening of hypoxia. I was deeply anxious that I might be ventilated anytime now. I was in the dark about the next step; all I knew was that my life had been turned upside down. The consultant in charge came in and said that in case there was no improvement, I might be ventilated that night.

My life had come to a standstill as the shadow of disease and death hung over me. I could feel the fear and at the same time I was determined not to be governed by fear and certainly not succumb to it.

Day 9

My wife, Arundhati, was very anxious. She was in the ward with Covid-19 infection although, fortunately, without much of lung involvement or hypoxia. My daughter lives in the USA, pursuing a fellowship in child and adolescent psychiatry. She got in touch with an immunologist she knew at Michigan University. He responded promptly and asked about the details of my case. His first reaction was that I required immediate high-dose steroids. Although I was getting Dexamethasone of 8mg twice daily, he said that the dosage was too low for such a high level of cytokine storm.

International Medical Board

Arundhati by then had contacted another critical care specialist in Philadelphia. These two Covid-19 specialists, along with the lady pulmonologist from another hospital in Kolkata and my consultant, agreed to set up an International Medical Board, with due permission from the Chairman of my hospital, who would be present along with my daughter in the USA and Arundhati.

I was completely unaware of all this. HFNO and prone breathing were going on to the best of my efforts. Plasma therapy and Remdesivir had not done me any good. After four hours, once the medical board's meeting was over, it was decided to withhold ventilation till a good dose of intravenous Methylprednisolone (steroid) was tried. There was some discussion about adding Favipiravir or Tocilizumab. The medical board very clearly spelled out that at that stage there was a cytokine storm and not much of primary viraemia after 10 days of onset of fever. Therefore, Favipiravir or even Tocilizumab would not work, rather my liver might suffer further damage and my condition might deteriorate. Medical literature about the use of Favipiravir and Tocilizumab after the 10th day of onset of first symptoms is mired in controversy. In fact, many scientific papers have shown no proven benefit of these drugs in treating Covid-19 patients.

Plasma therapy in the treatment of this disease has created a lot of buzz but of late the evidence of benefit has seemed doubtful. The US Food and Drug Administration (FDA) has not approved the routine use of plasma therapy in Covid-19 infection, and regulated it as an investigational product.

Day 10

At 1am on Day 10, 250mg intravenous Methylprednisolone — three times daily — along with high dose of antibiotics (Tazobactam, Piperacillin) was commenced. Arundhati and my daughter, Mishtoo (Dr Anindita Chakraborty), gave their consent for any risk caused by such a high dose of steroid. The immunologist from Michigan clearly stated that high-dose intravenous Methylprednisolone be started straightway. The critical care specialist and Covid doctor from Philadelphia was firm that at the critical stage I was in, high-dose steroid was the drug of choice. Later, a former colleague of mine from the UK was contacted and she endorsed the view. Another doctor from Perth, Australia, was also in agreement.

A key person on the medical board was the immunologist from Michigan, who was closely monitoring my condition and was in continuous touch with my primary consultant. The best thing was that all the clinicians from different parts of the world were in sync and in agreement. Everyone was truly and wholeheartedly supportive in steering me to the road to recovery. The hospital administration, especially the Chairman of the hospital, was extremely cooperative and was ensuring that the therapy continued as per the decisions of the medical board.

I was really fortunate to have such wonderful care, for which I am indebted to my wife, my daughter and of course to the very accomplished doctors of Kolkata, USA, UK and Australia.

I was happy that there was unanimous agreement regarding my treatment plan among my primary consultant, pulmonologist, immunologist from Michigan and critical care specialist from Philadelphia. They were all closely monitoring my progress to adjust my medication at every step.

Every week we are being attacked by dozens of viruses. But our body immune system fights them all. Medical literature has not shown that virus is being killed inside our body. In Covid-19 our body immune system while defending us against the virus creates a stormy chemical and cellular response which in some cases may be damaging and even deadly. This is the essence of pathology of the Covid-19 infection. To manage the cytokine tornado we need steroids and to prevent hypoxic damage we need adequate supply of oxygen.

By 10am of Day 10, I had received 2 doses of intravenous Methylprednisolone, altogether 500mg, along with 36 litre/minute of oxygen at 70 per cent fraction of inspired oxygen (FiO_2) through HFNO and prone position. By mid-day, the blood gas looked better. Clinically, oxygen saturation improved to 94 per cent and my breathing pattern improved. Anticoagulants, saline infusion, lung nebulizers and other drugs like antibiotics were going on as usual. By evening, the oxygen requirement reduced to 20 litre/min with 60 per cent FiO_2.

Was the worst, finally, over?

VIII

Remdesivir, Favipiravir, Tocilizumab, Plasma, Lenzilumab

As of November 2020, there is no well-established antiviral drug with proven efficacy for Covid-19 infection.

Remdesivir

Remdesivir is a broad-spectrum antiviral drug. It was tried in Ebola virus infection but there was limited benefit. It has been shown to inhibit the replication of coronavirus in tissue culture in severe acute respiratory infection (SARS) in 2003 and also in Middle East Respiratory Syndrome (MERS) in 2012.

The benefit of Remdesivir in treating Covid-19 infection has not yet been established. From various studies of small groups of patients, it has been observed that there may be clinical improvement in about 68 per cent of Covid-19 patients but at the same time in about 13 to 15 per cent patients there was mortality, more so when they were on ventilator. There are also reports of adverse effects like rise of liver enzymes, kidney damage and drop in blood pressure. Clearly, a lot of caution is to be taken while patients are on Remdesivir.

This drug was recommended initially by the US FDA as

emergency usage authorisation therapy, in the early stage of infection. In late October 2020, the FDA approved its use in some cases of Covid-19 during the early stage of infection in order to try and avoid hospitalisation. Some recent publications have shown no improvement of mortality in Covid-19 infection with the use of Remdesivir.

Favipiravir

Information about the use of Favipiravir and Tocilizumab in Covid-19 is inadequate. Efficacy and safety of Favipiravir for treatment of the virus has not yet been established. There is some information from China on the use of Favipiravir in Covid-19 showing marginal improvement. Furthermore, this drug has side effects like liver damage and others, which could be a big concern in patients.

Information about Lopinavir, Ritonavir is inadequate as of October 2020.

Tocilizumab

Tocilizumab is a monoclonal antibody. It blocks the cytokine IL-6 and may also prevent the genetic copying of the Covid-19 virus, thus blocking its reproduction. The evidence of Tocilizumab is conflicting. One study showed it reducing the likelihood of Covid-19 patients needing mechanical ventilation to about 44 per cent; but the mortality or discharge rate after 28 days was not found to be different for patients on or off Tocilizumab. Some more trials were not quite supportive of the use of this drug. Tocilizumab may be helpful in a small number of Covid-19 infections with a high level of inflammatory markers, a progressively rising requirement of oxygen and lung damage. However, there are a lot of side effects like complex bacterial and fungal infections. So, routine use of Tocilizumab has not yet been recommended.

Ivermectin

Ivermectin is an antiparasitic drug. In experimental laboratory setting, it has been shown to prevent the growth of RNA virus, like the one that causes Covid-19. But the effective dose required inside the human body to inhibit the growth of the Covid-19 virus is still unknown.

There has been talk of Ivermectin being some sort of a "cure" for Covid-19, when administered with the common antibiotic Doxycycline and zinc supplements. But there is no proper clinical study to support that. Such information is based on some clinicians' opinion or personal observation. Medical studies are unlikely to provide the high-quality data necessary to back these claims about the benefits of Ivermectin.

Plasma Therapy

In plasma therapy, people who have recovered from the disease donate their blood which has the antibodies to SARS-CoV-2 — the novel coronavirus that causes Covid-19.

The blood is processed to remove blood cells, leaving behind plasma and antibodies. This plasma is then transfused into an infected coronavirus patient to boost the ability to fight the virus.

Convalescent plasma therapy did not show significant benefit in reducing mortality risk among Covid-19 patients, according to an interim analysis of a randomised controlled trial conducted at the All India Institute of Medical Sciences (AIIMS), Delhi. Plasma therapy may have some role in the early stage of the disease. But for plasma therapy to be effective, the plasma must contain a sufficient amount of neutralising immunoglobulin IgG antibody against the Covid-19 virus spike protein.

Preparation of Covid convalescent plasma is different from that of conventional plasma preparation. This therapy also carries risks such as inadvertent transfer of blood-borne infections and reactions to serum constituents, including immunological reactions such as serum sickness, that may worsen the clinical condition of the patient. In addition, once some organs are damaged because of Covid-19, those might not recover after plasma therapy.

It is still unclear whether convalescent plasma will be an effective therapy for Covid-19. Despite little evidence of benefit, the US FDA has approved its use as emergency usage authorisation in hospitalised Covid-19 patients as an investigational drug. An authority like the Indian Council of Medical Research (ICMR), in its randomised controlled PLACID trial, has found that convalescent plasma did not forestall disease progression or even death.

Lenzilumab (Regeneron)

A descriptive analysis of Regeneron Pharmaceuticals' Phase I/II/III clinical trial has found that its antibody cocktail REGN-COV2 lowered viral load and reduced the time taken for symptoms improvement in non-hospitalised Covid-19 patients. It was developed for treatment of leukaemia and has also been tried in uncontrolled rheumatoid arthritis and advanced asthma. However, their clinical data in Covid-19 infection is only from 275 patients, of which there were some adverse effects. Lenzilumab has already been approved for the Ebola virus. Theoretically it may reduce the cytokine response of Covid-19, but we need to have more evidence. The US FDA has not yet approved it, as of early November 2020, although the company has submitted for acceptance.

Solidarity Trial

As released on October 15, 2020, the interim results of the Solidarity therapeutics trial — the largest international randomised trial of the WHO in 12,000 patients of at least 30 countries — did not show any mortality benefit or reduction of ventilation usage or decrease in hospital stay with the use of Remdesivir, Hydroxychloroquine, Lopinavir, Ritonavir or even Interferon in Covid-19 infection.

Steroid Therapy in Covid-19 Patients

Covid-19 has been known to the scientific community for less than nine months as of October 2020. The trajectory of the Covid-19 disease process remains mysterious. Clearly, much is yet to be understood, and the challenge for the near future will be to increase our understanding of the physiopathology of this novel infectious disease. The advances in our comprehension of the mechanisms sustaining the clinical course and patient-related factors driving the final outcome are vital to developing effective preventive strategies and/or therapeutical options.

Based on current knowledge, the cytokine storm is one of the most dangerous and potentially life-threatening events related to Covid-19. The immune-mediated events related to the response to this infection and the role of the cytokine/ chemokine receptor system are essential determinants for further and more extensively characterised understanding in order to identify targeted therapeutic strategies. Only from May-June 2020 have we understood that steroid therapy plays a key role to improve survival in critical infection. From medical literature, steroid therapy has proved to be effective in critical and severe Covid-19. In fact, it might be life-saving.

The hide-and-seek challenge game between the virus and our immune defences is intriguing. Perhaps this would help us understand the extremely variable spectrum of clinical manifestations of Covid-19, which appear to range from asymptomatic cases to lethal bilateral pneumonia with multi-organ failure and fatality. Such interaction may affect the brain, causing brain blood vessel disease displaying neuropsychiatric features such as incoherent talk, lack of insight, insomnia. It may affect the gastrointestinal system producing pain in the belly with distension, diarrhoea. At times it may cause kidney injury and affect the heart causing severe heart muscle disease myocarditis, arrhythmias, or heart failure which may be fatal.

Invasive Mechanical Ventilation in Covid-19 Patients

Many experts argued in February and March of 2020 that mechanical ventilation should be employed early in order to prevent Covid-19 patients progressing from mild disease to more severe lung injury. This viewpoint has been expressed most forcefully in a Journal of American Medical Association (JAMA) editorial, where authors attested that vigorous, spontaneous inspiration efforts can rapidly lead to self-induced lung injury. Early invasive mechanical ventilation would prevent this damage and save lives, it was argued. An insufficient supply of ventilators was feared, and some authorities even recommended connecting four patients to a single ventilator.

Looking at the projected number of Covid-19 patients worldwide, the fear of ventilator shortage prompted panicky politicians to urge automakers to branch into ventilator manufacture.

But with time and better understanding of the nature

of this disease, we have realised that the true impact of mechanical ventilation will never be known. It depends on whether intubated patients truly required mechanical ventilation or whether they could have been sustained with oxygen supplied by less drastic methods.

A good number of Covid-19 patients can be managed with supplemental oxygen, by HFNO along with drugs such as high-dose steroids. Patients with the most severe respiratory failure need insertion of an endotracheal tube. An endotracheal tube facilitates control over an unstable airway and enables precise regulation of oxygen, pressure and volume. But the endotracheal tube brings in its wake a slew of complications. Each day of mechanical ventilation exposes the patient to complications and increases mortality. Lung damage has been observed in some patients on invasive ventilation. Also, barotrauma (caused by high-pressure oxygen through ventilator) has been an independent risk factor.

Early ventilation may not help patients and, instead, steer things in the wrong direction. We should try to avoid invasive mechanical ventilation; rather, we should utilise HFNO and other non-invasive ventilation at the early stage of respiratory failure from Covid-19. Invasive ventilation should be reserved for a patient not improving despite all the above being tried and when the respiratory failure is getting worse. At that stage, ventilation is inevitable.

Extracorporeal Membrane Oxygenation (ECMO) and Covid-19

In Covid-19 patients, ECMO may represent an efficient support in case of severe and refractory respiratory dysfunction and/or cardiogenic/septic shock unresponsive to maximal therapy. Reports available as of October 2020 focusing on respiratory compromise treatment in Covid-19 patients and in particular those undergoing vein-to- vein ECMO therapy, however, are very restrained in declaring benefit. In medical literature, the information about the benefits of ECMO in severe respiratory failure with extensive pneumonia secondary to this infection is contradictory.

In Covid-19 infection, there are significant haematological and coagulation disorders, which may cause severe complications when these patients are put on ECMO support. ECMO itself may trigger inflammation and jeopardise the coagulation system, and so the already present hyper-inflammation of the cytokine storm of Covid-19 may further pull the patient down, with even fatal complications.

As much as possible, ECMO support should be deferred unless absolutely essential. Early introduction of ECMO might even be fatal. ECMO is helpful in a minuscule percentage of very critical Covid patients.

IX

Days 11, 12 and 13

On Day 11, my oxygen requirement came down to 10 litre/min with 50 per cent flow rate. Mentally I was alert, but my cough continued with a lot of thick mucus, and chest spasm. By this time, I was adopting the prone position quite comfortably. There was no discomfort with the HFNO tube sitting tight on my nose. Dryness in nasal cavities was managed well by saline wash.

Intravenous steroid in the same dosage was going on along with Enoxaparin, Apixaban, antibiotics and nebulisers containing steroid and bronchodilators. The blood reports of Day 11 were satisfactory. CRP, ferritin, D-dimer, IL-6 had come down. Kidney function, sodium and potassium were normal. Liver enzymes were raised but less than before. I continued to remain in a positive frame of mind. I was obdurate that by all means I must come out of this unprecedented medical crisis.

On Day 12, I was better. I could talk clearly. With clinical improvements, the chances of ventilation had of course gone down. Oxygen requirement came down further at 6-8 litre/min with 40 per cent FiO2 with HFNO. Cough and breathlessness were much less. Bronchial spasm had diminished, although I was on antispasmodic drugs. Blood gas reports showed the oxygen content of blood improving. I could manage to sit on a chair while on oxygen. I could communicate clearly. My personal hygiene was efficiently managed by attending nurses and the housekeeping team.

Day 13 was a much better day. I was on HFNO, the oxygen was at 6 litre/min with 35 per cent FiO2. My pulmonologist said that I was definitely improving. In fact, I should be able to switch over to the Venturi mask by evening, from HFNO, depending upon the blood gas report and oxygen flow requirements. I was out of my bed, and on a chair, comfortably. Some chest physiotherapy was going on. My appetite was good, the cough and the chest spasm were far less.

Blood was sent for all parameters. Blood gas analysis showed improvement of PO2 to 64 mmHg, PCO2 was 40 mmHg. HFNO was disconnected and I was put on a Venturi mask at 6 litre/min oxygen with 35 per cent FiO2. I slept the whole night in a prone position. Saturation remained at 97 per cent. The morning ICU nurse was very optimistic and assured me that eventually I would be able to go home. ICU is far from the natural world. I must get out of here, I kept telling myself.

Day 14

I woke up in the morning and felt fresh for the first time since I had come into the ICU. I rinsed my mouth while sitting on the chair next to the bed. I had breakfast. The ICU doctor and other staff were very happy to see me comfortable. Oxygen saturation was 97 per cent on 35 per cent Venturi mask with 6 litre/minute of oxygen flow. Intravenous

Methylprednisolone of 250mg, three times, was on. This was the fifth day on that dosage and from the next day it would come down to 250mg, twice daily.

I expressed my growing anxiety of staying on in the ICU. Every night some patients there were dying. Patients on ECMO were very critical. I was frightened every night. It made me emotionally exhausted.

Blood gas and other tests were sent. My primary consultant assured me that if the reports were satisfactory, I might be transferred back to the room by evening. However, even if I was taken to the room on the 6th floor, the ICU nurses would take care of me and there would be a continuous bedside monitor.

The blood gas reports were normal. The other reports came by afternoon. Clearly all inflammatory markers were significantly diminished. Oxygen saturation was 97-98 per cent on 5-6 litre/min flow rate with 35 per cent Venturi mask. My consultant came around 4pm. He had a discussion with other members of the critical care team and also the Chairman of the hospital. The decision was to transfer me to the room with ICU nursing support, bedside commode and bedside monitor.

It was great news for me. Arundhati was also on the 6th floor. Her Covid infection was less intense and was being treated in the ward. She was stable with saturation of 97 per cent without oxygen support. The good news went to her that I was a lot better and would be transferred out of the ICU by evening. What a relief for both of us.

Thoughts of a doctor lying helpless in ICU as a morbid patient

I was kept in a small room inside the 10-bed ICU. All patients, like myself, were critical. Three to four were on ventilators. On top of that, at least four patients were on ECMO. Every night, some very sick patients from other hospitals were being brought in for ECMO care.

I am an interventional cardiologist. I am very familiar with the precise meaning of the multiple sounds emanating from the monitors connected with patients. By listening to those sounds, I become acutely aware of what is wrong with a patient's vital parameters. The first two days, I was not in a condition to comprehend. But from day three of my ICU stay, when mentally I was more alert, I could listen to the heart rhythms of other patients and even the hushed discussions among doctors and nurses about the criticality of some patients. It was dreadful!

I could visualise that some patient near me was having a cardiac arrest. Some were just breathing their last. A ghastly thought gripped my mind. It was as if I was waiting in a queue and at any moment, I might have cardio-respiratory arrest. I would be resuscitated by the critical team and connected with a ventilator, and then I would be on for ECMO.

An interventional cardiologist was lying helpless as a critical Covid patient in the ICU. I could see, I could hear, I could fathom the morbid scenarios. At the same time, I was thinking how anyone's time in this world was a story of minutes.

There would be a lot of condolences, a flood of RIP (Rest in Peace) messages on WhatsApp. Family members would observe a period of grief for three to six months. But the world would not change. Nature would not change. The immortality of a soul would continue to be questioned. These thoughts kept hammering into my being, causing intense psychological turmoil. Amidst the cumulative fears from the sights and sounds around me, I was clear in my mind that I must move out of the ICU and back to the ward.

At the same time, I was acutely aware of the dedication and commitment that the ICU nurses had for their patients. It was amazing to witness how dutifully they were administering all the injections on time, drawing blood samples, taking care of all ventilated patients so efficiently. They were very polite, always supportive for all critical patients. The nurses, housekeeping, technical staff were always encouraging me. Despite my very critical condition I had regular injections of confidence that I would be able to come out of this crisis.

In three shifts there were three male nurses, brothers as they called themselves. They were really very well trained. They had the skills and the aptitude to handle all the equipment in the ICU. The HFNO machine is a kind of new machine, mostly used for Covid patients. At times the saline flow was improper, or the tubes and propellers were not fitted well. These brothers could correct those flaws competently. It was really very impressive. At times their knowledge of ICU care appeared better than that of junior doctors! With their continued support and assistance, even during my worst phase, I was motivated to push myself towards recovery.

Needless to say, doctors, nurses and people working in healthcare are particularly vulnerable to this highly infectious disease. In response to the global pandemic, the under-resourced doctors are facing unprecedented challenges. In many hospitals, Covid wards do not have enough staff or even round-the-clock doctors on site.

The list of our sleep-deprived heroes includes doctors, nurses, medical cleaners, pathologists, paramedics, ambulance drivers and healthcare administrators. In the fight against the coronavirus, the brave medical army stands strong with thermometers, stethoscopes and ventilators as their weapons. Not to forget the medical researchers who are working day and night against all odds, hoping to find the antidote to this deadly disease. Since the coronavirus outbreak, healthcare professionals have not only experienced the gratification of patients healed and lives saved but they have also lost many battles along the way. On top of that, many doctors have sacrificed their own lives in the line of duty. Such loss is reprehensible. Every day, every night, these selfless healthcare warriors are giving it their all while cutting themselves off from their families and loved ones. The sacrifice that they are making for the safety and welfare of humanity is priceless and deserves lifelong gratitude from us. Most importantly, we must reassess the value healthcare workers hold in our lives and the kind of treatment that they get from society.

Among the several lessons this coronavirus pandemic has been teaching us, the biggest one is to find ways to sufficiently invest in better and more efficient medical facilities and give medical professionals the respect, compensation and infrastructure that they truly deserve. Moreover, the world needs to work towards advancement in medical research and technology. Nothing will be a greater tribute to the healthcare fraternity than this. I must acknowledge with the highest sense of gratitude the heroic efforts of the courageous and inspirational doctors from across the globe who have lost their lives while saving the lives of Covid-19 patients.

Recovery from ICU

On the evening of Day 14, after I returned to the 6th floor room, I felt reassured to a great extent. First thing, I looked at the sky through the window. It was a dark evening with scattered clouds, peeping stars and a glitter of lights. I lay in bed, mostly in a prone position. Oxygen was flowing at 6 litre/min with 35 per cent Venturi mask. Intravenous saline infusion was on. Antibiotics, steroid, anticoagulants, bronchodilators were continuing. The ICU male nurses (brothers) were with me round the clock. They were there to arrange my bed, help me use the commode, have a wash, maintain oral hygiene, and they did it all with a pleasant demeanour and an encouraging spirit. Their commitment to their job was outstanding.

Day 15 to Day 24

I had a sound sleep and woke up early on the morning of Day 15. I saw sunrise — after around 10 days — through the window panes of my room. Inside the ICU, I could not differentiate between day and night. I was in a small, closed room which was always illuminated with lamps as is the norm in ICU wards. My biological clock was haywire. Back in my room, looking at the daylight outside, I felt rejuvenated. I could see green trees, wide roads, flow of traffic, just another busy day of human life!

On Day 15 and Day 16, I remained on 35 per cent Venturi mask with oxygen flow of 5-6 litre/min. Steroid dosage was reduced to 125mg three times daily. I remained in a prone position for at least 14 hours during these two days. On Day 16, blood was sent for tests. Supportive care such as chest physiotherapy, limb movements, care for bladder and bowel functions were provided proficiently by staff from physiotherapy. Blood reports showed improvement. I was happy with the progress.

On Day 17 and Day 18, oxygen saturation was 96-98 per cent with 4 litre/min of oxygen. Venturi mask was changed to 28 per cent. From Day 19, I was mobile. I started walking inside the room for at least six minutes, slowly. Most of the day, I spent sitting on a chair. I was able to comfortably eat breakfast, lunch and dinner. From Day 20, the special ICU nurses left me in the care of scheduled nurses of the ward. The sister in charge of the 6th floor Covid ward was incredible. She took excellent and personal care of me and Arundhati.

Arundhati was very anxious all along. In addition, steroid therapy (although at a lower dose than mine) and may be the Covid infection itself made her very irritable. Her sleep pattern was severely disturbed. She required some psychiatry consultation and was prescribed a small dose of short-term antipsychotic drugs. Fortunately, she recovered within a short period. Neuropsychiatry manifestations of Covid-19 infection are being well documented.

From Day 20, I was able to go to the toilet on my own. Intravenous drugs were discontinued. The steroid dose was changed to oral tablets, 80mg Prednisolone twice daily, antibiotics were changed to oral tablets, Enoxaparin injection was discontinued. Oxygen requirement was about 2-3 litre/min through simple nasal cannula. From Day 21, I was able to walk in the corridor of the ward without any support. Physiotherapy was going on regularly. My consultant started planning for discharge.

However, as my oxygen requirement was very high (more than 15 litre/minute), it was mandatory by local government regulations that I must be Covid negative before discharge. On Day 22, RTPCR (Reverse transcriptase polymerase chain reaction) was done. It turned out to be positive. I was told that during the recovery phase of Covid infection, RTPCR might be positive if some dead viral fragments remain hanging around the nasal and oral cavities. But I was not infective. A repeat test was planned after two days. A negative test would allow me to go home. Otherwise I might have to stay on a bit longer.

The blood tests of Day 23 were normal. All parameters of inflammation had reached normal levels. There was some rise of neutrophil count with less lymphocytes, most likely because of steroid therapy. Clinically I was up and about. I had no fever, no cough, no spasm, no breathlessness. On Day 23 and 24, I was on 1.5-2 litre/min of oxygen through ordinary nasal cannula. This was as good as being in room air.

Day 25

It was a bright, sunny morning. At 7am a senior sister from the ward came in and took swabs for RTPCR. I was cheerful and had no discomfort. There was hardly any oxygen requirement. Saturation was maintained at 96-97 per cent off oxygen. At 2pm of Day 25, my Covid-19 report came in. I was negative for the virus as per RTPCR. I was finally ready to head home.

The paperwork was being processed, and it would take about four to five hours before I could physically leave the hospital. Arundhati had been discharged three days earlier. She was, however, staying on as my attendant. Both of us were told very clearly that although we were medically fit to go home, it was extremely important to take adequate rest. Physiotherapy and rehabilitation must be followed properly. It would take me at least two full months for complete recovery.

XI

Covid, Other Organs, and the Mind

Other than the lungs, Covid is known to also affect the brain, heart, belly, liver, kidney. The primary cause is blood vessel damage of these vital organs. Direct heart involvement is rare, but in some cases there might be damage to heart muscles even a month into recovery. Fortunately, my other organs have remained least affected.

Preliminary reports concerning the psychological health effects of Covid-19 include acute stress associated with symptom progression and severe distress during ICU treatment (for example, nightmares and extreme fear that frequently occur with delirium). In addition, there may be fear of death, delirium, and concern about family and friends, contributing to persistent symptoms of anxiety, depression, post-traumatic stress disorder (PTSD) and fatigue over months or even years.

About one out of three survivors who required hospitalisation might suffer long-lasting emotional problems. A psychiatrist or a psychologist may be of great help to deal with this. For some patients, a short course of antipsychotic drugs or anxiolytic medicines has been found to be very effective.

In some patients there may be persistent muscle pain

and muscular weakness. I had similar symptoms, more of muscular weakness than pain. This was attributed to high dose steroid therapy.

Rehabilitation

Critically ill Covid-19 survivors may experience a wide range of sequels, resulting in long-lasting physical, cognitive, and psychological dysfunction. Early rehabilitation can mitigate these complications and improve the quality of life. Rehabilitation is the key to ensure that patients do not deteriorate after discharge and require readmission.

Patients with Covid-19 have a need for rehabilitation during and directly after hospitalisation. Physical and mental rehabilitation professionals are frontline healthcare professionals and should be engaged in the care of patients suffering from severe cases of Covid-19. In fact, rehabilitation starts even when the patient is in hospital — either in the ward or in the critical care unit. Rehabilitation in the ICU helps improve the functional ability of patients. Early mobilisation is very important. Proper leg and arm physiotherapy along with lung function improvement by chest physiotherapy are essential. In addition, psychological support for these patients improves their alertness, cognitive functions and mental stability. All this rehabilitation for Covid patients must be continued long after discharge to enable them to get back to a pre-infection quality of life soon.

Long Haul Covid-19

It has been found that in about 20% of Covid-19 patients between 20-38 years of age, some symptoms like cough, malaise, weakness, muscle pain continue even 2 to 6 months after recovery. In patients above 60 years the figure may be as high as 35-45%. These are called long haul Covid patients. The exact mechanism of persistence of these symptoms is unclear. Life as a long hauler can be scary, confusing and frustrating, especially for those who otherwise led a very active life before the illness.

A British Medical Journal and JAMA Research publication confirmed the existence of long haul Covid from patients who were treated in Italy. Tim Spector, professor of genetic epidemiology at King's College London, has shown that in 12% patients Covid symptoms persist for more than 30 days and in one out of 200 these may remain beyond 90 days. There is no specific treatment for this and apparently with time the symptoms cool down. But certainly for these patients adequate rest and avoidance of exertion are mandatory. Some of them may develop late onset cardiac arrhythmia, myocarditis, cerebral problems and cognitive disorders. These patients must remain under close supervision.

Prevention

Around 80 per cent of infected individuals remain asymptomatic and continue to spread the disease. No definitive and fail-proof treatment is available till date. The common routes of transmission, as mentioned earlier, are the droplets and close contact through air-borne influences. Sneezing, coughing, infected surface, etc, are transmission routes for Covid-19. The main strategy is to prevent spread from this super-spreader. Prevention is better than cure.

The most effective prevention to avoid spreading of Covid-19 is maintaining social distancing and hand hygiene, wearing masks, using sanitisers, avoiding handshakes or personal physical contact, and steering clear of all kinds of social gatherings.

Hydroxychloroquine has been widely used as a preventive therapy for Covid-19 infection, but its role to prevent the infection has not been established. The same is true for Ivermectin.

Vaccine

At the time of writing this, more than 150 coronavirus vaccines are in development across the world, and hopes are pinned on bringing some to market in record time to ease the global crisis. Several efforts are underway to help make that possible with a WHO-led aim to deliver two billion doses by the end of 2021.

A vaccine goes through clinical trials over three stages before reaching regulatory agencies for approval, which can be a lengthy process by itself.

After a vaccine is approved, it faces the challenges of where and who, how many and at what cost when it comes to production and distribution. Many vaccines also stay in what's called "phase four" — a perpetual stage of regulatory study.

What does a Covid-19 vaccine aim to do? Like all vaccines, it essentially aims to instruct the immune system to mount a defence. To do so, some vaccines use the whole coronavirus, but in a killed or weakened state. Others use only part of the virus — whether a protein or a fragment. Some transfer the coronavirus proteins into a different virus that is unlikely to cause disease or is incapable of it. Finally, some vaccines under development rely on deploying pieces of the coronavirus's genetic material, so our cells can temporarily make the coronavirus proteins needed to stimulate our immune systems.

It is too early to say which vaccine will ultimately be successful, and when. However, Pfizer in collaboration with German company BioNTech, has developed a RNA based vaccine with more than 90% efficacy. This vaccine has to be preserved in minus 70° centigrade even during transportation which might be a challenge. Moderna Inc. of the USA has developed a vaccine which claims an efficacy of 95% against Covid-19. The preservation temperature is much simpler as compared to the Pfizer-BioNTech vaccine. These are promising.

The United Kingdom is the first western country to have started a mass vaccination programme against Covid-19, with Margaret Keenan, a 90-year-old lady of Coventry, becoming the first person to receive this vaccine outside the trial. In the USA, the Pfizer vaccine has already got FDA approval and Sandra Lindsay, a healthcare worker of New York, received the first vaccine of Pfizer-BioNTech there.

The vaccine of AstraZeneca, of Oxford University group, is coming out with promising protection and relatively simple preservation methods. In India, Covaxin of Bharat Biotech has generated a robust immune response with high neutralising antibodies. Simultaneously, vaccines are in development in Russia and China. The Russian vaccine is nearly ready for use.

Like any other vaccine, Covid vaccines may have some adverse reactions like mild allergic features, fever, joint pain, etc. But overall protection against the brutal bug is essential for the human community. An active vaccination programme is in the process of being launched worldwide.

Initial results from trials and even from clinical applications are promising and I am hopeful that by March-April 2021, people of this world will largely be protected by active vaccination against the deadly Covid-19 pathogen.

Mutant Covid-19

When Covid-19 spread around the globe, researchers and medical scientists started speculating how the deadly virus might be changing its character as it passed from person to person. A new study published in *Science* confirms that SARS-CoV-2 has mutated in a way that's enabled it to spread quickly.

A mutation means a change in the genetic sequence of the virus. In the case of SARS-CoV-2, which is an RNA virus, a mutation means a change in the sequence in which its molecules are arranged. A mutation in an RNA virus often happens when the virus makes a mistake while it is making copies of itself.

It has been observed that the mutant virus spreads faster. The transmission rate is as high as 70%. However the virulence of the mutant virus may not be as brawny as the original Covid-19.

Coronavirus vaccines are designed to create antibodies targeting the spike protein. Vaccines target multiple regions on the spike, while a mutation refers to a change in a single point. So, if there is one mutation, it does not mean vaccines would not work. The spike mutation may even make the virus more susceptible to a vaccine.

It is too early to comment on the nature of the mutant virus. We need to wait till we get more information about it. As of now we must continue to follow the standard protocols to prevent infection from Covid-19 and its mutants. Vaccination protocol should be followed.

XII

Homeward Bound

Finally, around 5pm on Day 25, I was officially discharged from hospital. The hospital Chairman visited us in the morning and was happy to see that we might be going home by evening depending upon my Covid report. My primary consultant, hospital medical superintendent, nursing in-charge of the 6th floor, all came at 5pm and greeted us with best wishes. That day also happened to be my birthday. The hospital authorities sent a nice cake for me. Being a Covid ward, there were a lot of restrictions. Despite that, all the nurses, doctors, housekeeping staff in their PPEs came to my room and had a small but very meaningful birthday celebration for 10 minutes. I felt delighted and grateful.

From a near-death experience, I was ready to go home. It was a great feeling. As if I was born again. By 630pm, the wheelchairs arrived inside the room. Arundhati and I were taken down to the main lobby where my primary consultant was waiting for us. I was touched. He repeatedly emphasised that I must take enough rest. I should continue physiotherapy. I must take my medicines on time. He insisted that we should contact him for any need at any time of day or night. He had ensured that all medicines would be procured on my way back home and had even arranged for an oxygen concentrator to be put in the boot of my car. Saying goodbye to everyone, Arundhati and I headed home.

After 25 days in the hospital, we were homeward bound. It seemed like the skyline had changed. Had the world also changed in these 25 days? The roads, the traffic, the lights, everything looked different. It was as if this was a colourful gift of life on my birthday. We were entering a new normal life. My heart was filled with gratitude for every staff of the hospital. I kept thinking of my debt to the Covid warriors while the car was navigating through this new normal city from the hospital to my home.

The memory of fighting Covid will remain with me as long as I exist on this planet. Covid-19 did shake the world like a health quake. It shook me too. But, finally, I won the battle. A tough time had ended, a good time was beginning.

I remembered how when I was inside the ICU as a critical patient, with death almost breathing down my neck, I did not give up. To remain alive was a challenge. Even when 36 litres of oxygen was flowing into me every minute and I was thinking in a clouded mental state that one of those breaths might be my last one, I was constantly fighting for life. Even at that stage, I tried to remain as strong as I mentally could so that I would win this battle. I did witness every night how many critical patients succumbed to death while they were either on the ventilator or ECMO.

Being a doctor, I never believed that such precious human lives could end in such a helpless manner. I could not understand why we, the medical community, were taking so long to fathom the intricate disease trajectory of Covid-19 infection when medicine has developed so much in the 21st century. It is so frustrating. The value of human life has been completely shattered in the face of the Covid-19 virus.

I have survived and emerged victorious. There is now a renewed urge inside me to save human lives from this venomous bug. It is my intense appeal that everyone must take all precautionary measures like wearing masks, using sanitisers, maintaining social distance and at the early onset of any kind of fever get a Covid-19 test done and go into self-isolation. If mildly symptomatic and Covid-19 positive, you may remain in self quarantine with close monitoring.

In the case of moderate to severe symptoms with positive tests, patients *must* get admitted in a Covid hospital after being seen by a Covid specialist. Early treatment with steroids after three to five days of fever in case there is a drop in oxygen saturation below 93 per cent is extremely helpful. Avoidance of mechanical ventilation does reduce mortality. Physicians and many healthcare workers need Covid education and updates about its management. This pandemic is destroying our world. We the survivors must do all that we can to save our own world.

The new world created by this horrible microbe is not the world that we would like to live in. Our world vibrates with joy, with happiness, with fun and lively colours. Covid-19 has snatched many lives from this world. But it will never snatch our lovely world from our lives. We the Covid survivors are committed to saving you from this cruel germ.

The Covid-19 pandemic is not a political chant. It is truly a terminator bug for human lives in this world. Medical scientists and doctors are dedicated souls, committed to maintaining the wellness of human life. I am a doctor. I returned to life from the brink of death. Perhaps my experience of battling this disease is an opportunity to offer Covid victims my insights and advice. In every decade in the history of medicine, human civilisation has faced challenges. Eventually, the medical community has succeeded in combating them. I am sure the tyranny of Covid-19 will also come to an end. And human life will continue to blossom.

Humanity will win, just like I did.

About the Author

Dr Rabin Chakraborty

MD (PGIMER, Chandigarh), DNB, MRCP, FRCP (London), FRCP (Glasgow), FRCP (Ireland), FACC (USA), FICC, FISE, FICP, FCSI, DM (Cardiology, PGIMER, Chandigarh)

A Senior Consultant Interventional Cardiologist & Electrophysiologist, Dr Chakraborty is Senior Vice Chairman, Cardiology Services, Medica Group of Hospitals.

He is also Examiner MRCP (UK), Examiner, National Board, DNB, the Cardiology President Elect, Indian College of Cardiology, the Associate Editor, *Journal of Indian Medical Association* (JIMA), and Chairperson, Health Committee, The Bengal Chamber of Commerce & Industry.

Formerly Consultant Cardiologist and Electrophysiologist, Hull Royal Infirmary and Castle Hill Hospital, East Yorkshire NHS trust, England, UK. Formerly Regional Director and Head of Cardiology, Apollo Gleneagles Hospitals, Kolkata. He conducts free health camps in villages, schools and orphanages

He has more than 75 publications in International Journals and is the author of two books on ECG for General Practitioners and medical students.

A man of letters, he has also published two books of poetry.

www.ingramcontent.com/pod-product-compliance
Lightning Source LLC
Chambersburg PA
CBHW030951240526
45463CB00016B/2484